Table of Contents

Introduction

Potassium is a mineral required by the body for several physiological processes including regulating heart function, fluid balance, and plays a role in nerve conduction and muscle contraction. Since your body cannot make potassium itself, it requires an external source, your food to obtain it.

Maintaining the right balance of potassium in the body is key. Too much or too little potassium can cause unwanted effects.

If the potassium in your blood is too low (this is called hypokalemia) you may experience weakness, fatigue, muscle cramps and/or abnormal heart beats.

If your potassium becomes too high (this is called hyperkalemia) you may experience nausea, vomiting, weakness, muscle fatigue, irregular heartbeat and/or paralysis. In severe cases high potassium can cause death. To maintain this delicate balance your body primarily uses its kidneys to regulate potassium.

There are several reasons why you could need a low potassium diet. The most common reason is a decline of kidney function called chronic kidney disease (CKD). Other reasons for high potassium in the blood are Addison's disease, and use of certain medications.

If you have any conditions that put you at risk for high potassium levels, you doctor should be monitoring you with regular blood work. If you show signs of high potassium, your doctor will then recommend you follow a low potassium diet. It is usually not recommended to start a low potassium diet until you need to, that is until your blood shows abnormally high levels of potassium. In early stages of kidney disease, with only a slight decline in kidney function, it is not always necessary to worry about potassium in your diet.

A low potassium diet is defined as one that limits dietary sources of potassium to 2,000mg per day, which is just under half of what is recommended for the healthy population. That said, the degree to which you need to limit dietary potassium really depends on your individual kidney function, those with mild disease, it may not be necessary to strictly limit potassium.

Foods Contain Potassium

If you have been put on a low potassium diet and done some of your own research, you will quickly realize that potassium is in many foods. And not just that, it is in all the healthy foods that you thought you should be eating. Fruits and vegetables, nuts and seeds, legumes, dairy, and whole grains are all sources of potassium. The good news is that each one of these food groups contains foods with varying levels of potassium, so while you may need to limit certain fruits or vegetables, for example, there are many others that you can enjoy.

Upon learning that potassium is in so many foods, it's not uncommon to feel overwhelmed. This is another reason why consulting with a Registered Dietitian or Renal Dietitian is in your favour. They can help sort out what foods are the highest sources and help you put some reasonable limits on those higher potassium foods.

For those with quite low kidney function, potassium restriction must be more strictly followed. Additionally, anyone who may need to be mindful of their potassium intake for other reasons, may require varying degrees of dietary restriction. This is why the help of an experienced Registered Dietitian or Renal Dietitian (aka a Kidney Dietitian) is key. A Dietitian can help you figure out which level of potassium restriction is required for you, at this point in your life.

Fruits:

• Avocado

• Banana

• Citrus fruits (grapefruit, orange, tangerine, lemons, limes, etc.)

• Dried fruits

• Honeydew

Milk and Dairy Products:

• All milks (whole, 2%, 1%, skim)

Vegetables:

• Baked beans

• Brussel sprouts

• Carrots

• Greens (except kale & lettuce)

• Parsnips

• Spinach

• Squash (acorn, hubbard, butternut)

Acceptable Food Choices

Fruits:

• Apples, apple juice, applesauce

• Berries

• Fruit cocktail

• Peaches

• Pears

• Pineapple or pineapple juice

• Plums

Milk and Dairy Products:

• Cheddar or Swiss Cheese

• Low fat Cottage Cheese

Meats, Poultry, Fish, Dried Beans, Peas, Eggs:

• Chicken

• Turkey

• Eggs

• Shrimp

Vegetables:

• Asparagus

• Beans (green or yellow)

• Broccoli

• Cooked carrots

• Cauliflower

- Kale

- Lettuce

- Mushrooms

- Peas

- Peppers

Recipes

Apple Stuffed Pork Chops

Servings: 6

Yield: 6 chops

Ingredients

- 1 tablespoon chopped onion

- ¼ cup butter

- 3 cups fresh bread crumbs

- 2 cups chopped apples

- ¼ cup chopped celery

• 2 teaspoons chopped fresh parsley

• ¼ teaspoon salt

• 6 (1 1/4 inch) thick pork chops

• salt and pepper to taste

• 1 tablespoon vegetable oil

Instructions

• Preheat oven to 350 degrees F (175 degrees C).

• In a large skillet saute onion in butter or margarine until tender. Remove from heat. Add the bread crumbs, apples, celery, parsley and salt. Mix all together. Cut a large pocket in the side of each pork chop; season inside and out with salt and pepper to taste. Spoon apple mixture loosely into pockets.

• In skillet, heat oil to medium high and brown chops on both sides. Place browned chops in an ungreased 9x13 inch baking dish. Cover with aluminum foil and bake in the preheated oven for 30 minutes. Remove cover and bake for 30 minutes longer or until juices run clear.

Nutrition Facts Per Serving:

• 483 calories

• protein 32.2g

• carbohydrates 45g

• fat 18.9g

• cholesterol 89.7mg

• sodium 625.7mg

Angel Hair Pasta with Peppers and Chicken

Servings: 8

Yield: 8 servings

Ingredients

• 1 teaspoon olive oil

• 1 tablespoon minced garlic

• 1 large red bell pepper, julienned

• ¾ (8 ounce) can sliced water chestnuts

• 1 cup sugar snap pea pods

• 6 thick slices smoked deli chicken

• 1 tablespoon onion powder

• ¼ teaspoon ground black pepper

• 1 pinch salt

• 1 cup chicken broth

• 2 (8 ounce) packages angel hair pasta

Instructions

• In a large skillet, heat olive oil to medium high heat. Add the garlic, bell pepper, water chestnuts and pea pods. Reduce heat to medium low and cover. Cook for 5 minutes.

• Cut chicken into strips, approximately 1/4 inch wide. Add the chicken, onion powder, ground black pepper and salt to the skillet. Cover and cook for 5 more minutes.

• In a separate small saucepan, heat the chicken broth to a near boil. Pour the hot broth into the vegetable/chicken skillet. Toss and serve mixture over cooked angel hair pasta immediately.

Nutrition Facts Per Serving:

- 222 calories

- protein 10.7g

- carbohydrates 38.2g

- fat 2.8g

- cholesterol 10.1mg

- sodium 368.6mg

Italian Pasta Salad I

Prep: 15 mins

Cook: 15 mins

Total: 30 mins

Servings: 12

Yield: 12 servings

Ingredients

- 1 (16 ounce) package rotini pasta

- 1 cup Italian-style salad dressing

- 1 cup creamy Caesar salad dressing

- 1 cup grated Parmesan cheese

- 1 red bell pepper, diced

- 1 green bell pepper, chopped

- 1 red onion, diced

Instructions

- In a large pot of salted boiling water, cook pasta until al dente, rinse under cold water and drain.

- In a large bowl, combine the pasta, Italian salad dressing, Caesar dressing, Parmesan cheese, red bell pepper, green bell pepper, and red onion. Mix well and serve chilled or at room temperature.

Nutrition Facts Per Serving:

- 291 calories

- protein 8.5g

- carbohydrates 32.6g

- fat 14.6g

- cholesterol 5.9mg

• sodium 728.2mg

Prep: 15 mins

Cook: 15 mins

Total: 30 mins

Servings: 8

Yield: 8 servings

Ingredients

• 1 (16 ounce) package uncooked linguine pasta

• 2 tablespoons olive oil

• ¾ cup butter

• 3 cloves garlic, chopped

• 2 tablespoons fresh thyme leaves

• 5 roasted red peppers, drained and coarsely chopped

Instructions

• Bring a large pot of lightly salted water to a boil. Add linguine and olive oil, cook for 8 to 10 minutes, until al dente, and drain.

• Melt 2 tablespoons butter in a saucepan over medium heat. Stir in garlic, and cook until golden brown. Mix in remaining butter, thyme, and roasted red peppers. Continue to cook and stir until heated through. Serve over the cooked pasta.

Nutrition Facts Per Serving:

• 405 calories

• protein 7.9g

• carbohydrates 43.9g

• fat 22g

• cholesterol 45.8mg

• sodium 379.1mg

Easy Tuna Casserole

Prep: 15 mins

Cook: 30 mins

Total: 45 mins

Servings: 8

Yield: 8 servings

Ingredients

- 3 cups cooked macaroni

- 1 (5 ounce) can tuna, drained

- 1 (10.75 ounce) can condensed cream of chicken soup

- 1 cup shredded Cheddar cheese

- 1 ½ cups French fried onions

Instructions

- Preheat oven to 350 degrees F (175 degrees C).

- In a 9x13-inch baking dish, combine the macaroni, tuna, and soup. Mix well, and then top with cheese.

- Bake at 350 degrees F (175 degrees C) for about 25 minutes, or until bubbly. Sprinkle with fried onions, and bake for another 5 minutes. Serve hot.

Nutrition Facts Per Serving:

- 462 calories

- protein 11.5g

- carbohydrates 37.1g

- fat 28.5g

- cholesterol 22.6mg

- sodium 705.8mg

Tomatoless Pizza

Prep: 15 mins

Cook: 15 mins

Total: 30 mins

Servings: 4

Yield: 4 servings

Ingredients

- 1 (10 ounce) can refrigerated pizza crust dough

- 1 cup light sour cream

- 1 cup light cream cheese, softened

- 1 teaspoon dried dill weed

- 1 tablespoon olive oil

- 5 fresh mushrooms, sliced

- 1 small onion, peeled and sliced

- 1 clove garlic, minced

- ½ red bell pepper, seeded and sliced into strips

- ¾ cup baby spinach leaves

Instructions

- Preheat the oven to 375 degrees F (190 degrees C).

- Unroll the pizza dough onto a greased baking sheet. Press out to cover the entire sheet. In a medium bowl, mix together the sour cream, cream cheese and dill until smooth. Spread evenly over the crust.

- Heat the olive oil in a skillet over medium heat. Add the onion, mushrooms, garlic and red bell pepper; cook and stir until onion is tender but the pepper is still crisp, about 4 minutes. Stir in baby spinach at the end of cooking. Spread this mixture over the top of the pizza.

• Bake for 15 minutes in the preheated oven, or until the crust is golden at the edges. Cut into squares to serve.

Nutrition Facts Per Serving:

• 403 calories

• protein 17.1g

• carbohydrates 49.2g

• fat 15g

• cholesterol 39.9mg

• sodium 873.2mg

Rice with Herbes de Provence

Prep: 2 mins

Cook: 23 mins

Total: 25 mins

Servings: 4

Yield: 4 servings

Ingredients

• 1 cup white rice

• 2 cups chicken stock

• 1 ½ teaspoons herbes de Provence

• 1 pinch sea salt

• 1 pinch pepper

Instructions

• In a medium saucepan stir together rice, chicken stock, herbes de Provence, salt, and pepper. Set over high heat, and bring to a simmer; cover, and cook 20 minutes.

• Fluff with a fork, and serve.

Nutrition Facts Per Serving:

• 169 calories

• protein 3.3g

• carbohydrates 37.1g

• fat 0.3g

• sodium 82.4mg

Pear and Prosciutto Pizza

Prep: 25 mins

Cook: 45 mins

Total: 1 hr 10 mins

Servings: 4

Yield: 1 pizza

Ingredients

• 6 cloves garlic

• ½ tablespoon olive oil

• 2 ripe pears, halved and cored

• 1 tablespoon olive oil

• all-purpose flour for dusting

• 1 unbaked pizza crust

• 1 tablespoon cornmeal for dusting

• 6 ounces shredded Swiss cheese

• 5 thin slices prosciutto, cut into halves

• 1 (6 ounce) package fresh mozzarella, cut into small cubes

• salt and ground black pepper to taste

• ½ tablespoon olive oil

Instructions

• Preheat oven to 375 degrees F (190 degrees C). Place the garlic in a small square of aluminum foil. Drizzle 1/2 tablespoon of olive oil over the garlic. Wrap foil around garlic to seal.

• Roast the garlic in the preheated oven until soft, about 20 minutes. Smash roasted cloves with a fork.

• Place the pears in a bowl with 1 tablespoon olive oil; toss to coat. Arrange pear slices on a baking sheet.

• Bake in hot oven until soft, 10 to 15 minutes.

• Raise oven temperature to 400 degrees F (200 degrees C). Preheat a pizza stone or baking sheet in the oven.

• Lightly dust a flat surface with flour. Roll the prepared pizza crust dough out onto the prepared surface. Dust a baking sheet with cornmeal. Lay the dough onto the prepared baking sheet. Spread the mashed garlic onto the dough; top with the Swiss cheese. Arrange the pears, prosciutto, and mozzarella cheese onto the pizza. Season with salt and pepper. Brush the edges of the crust with the 1/2 tablespoon olive oil.

• Bake in preheated oven until the cheese is melted and crust is golden brown, 15 to 20 minutes.

Nutrition Facts Per Serving:

• 618 calories

• protein 30.6g

• carbohydrates 54.7g

• fat 30.7g

• cholesterol 73.8mg

• sodium 990mg

Pad Kee Mao

Prep: 20 mins

Cook: 20 mins

Additional: 1 hr

Total: 1 hr 40 mins

Servings: 4

Yield: 4 servings

Ingredients

• 3 ½ ounces dried Thai-style rice noodles, wide (such as Chantaboon Rice Noodles)

• 1 ½ teaspoons olive oil

• 2 cloves garlic, minced

• ½ teaspoon thick soy sauce

• 2 teaspoons white sugar

• 1 ½ teaspoons olive oil

• 2 cloves garlic, minced

• ½ pound pork (any cut), thinly sliced

• 1 serrano pepper, minced, or more to taste

• 30 fresh basil leaves, chopped

• ½ teaspoon thick soy sauce

• 1 teaspoon white sugar

• 1 teaspoon salt

• ½ cup bean sprouts

Instructions

• Place the dry rice noodles in a bowl, cover with hot water, and let soak until white and softened, about 1 hour. Drain the noodles, and set aside.

• Heat 1 1/2 teaspoon of olive oil in a wok or large skillet over low heat, and cook and stir 2 minced garlic cloves until brown and beginning to crisp, 2 to 3 minutes. Stir in the soaked noodles, 1/2 teaspoon of thick soy sauce, and 2 teaspoons of sugar, and cook and stir until the noodles have absorbed the soy sauce and turned brown, about 3 minutes. Remove the noodles from the skillet.

• Heat the remaining 1 1/2 teaspoons of olive oil in the wok over low heat; stir in the remaining 2 minced garlic cloves, and cook until brown and beginning to crisp, 2 to 3 minutes. Raise the heat to medium-high, and stir in the pork, serrano pepper, basil, 1/2 teaspoon thick soy sauce, 1 teaspoon sugar, and salt.

• Cook and stir until the pork is no longer pink and the edges of the meat are beginning to brown, about 5 minutes. Return the noodles to the wok, and stir in the bean sprouts.

• Cook and stir until heated through, about 5 more minutes.

Nutrition Facts Per Serving:

• 218 calories

• protein 7.2g

• carbohydrates 26.2g

• fat 9.1g

• cholesterol 22.3mg

• sodium 707.5mg

Apple Crisp II

Prep: 30 mins

Cook: 45 mins

Additional: 5 mins

Total: 1 hr 20 mins

Servings: 12

Yield: 1 9x13-inch pan

Ingredients

• 10 cups all-purpose apples, peeled, cored and sliced

• 1 cup white sugar

• 1 tablespoon all-purpose flour

• 1 teaspoon ground cinnamon

• ½ cup water

• 1 cup quick-cooking oats

• 1 cup all-purpose flour

• 1 cup packed brown sugar

- ¼ teaspoon baking powder

- ¼ teaspoon baking soda

- ½ cup butter, melted

Instructions

- Preheat oven to 350 degrees F (175 degree C).

- Place the sliced apples in a 9x13 inch pan. Mix the white sugar, 1 tablespoon flour and ground cinnamon together, and sprinkle over apples. Pour water evenly over all.

- Combine the oats, 1 cup flour, brown sugar, baking powder, baking soda and melted butter together. Crumble evenly over the apple mixture.

- Bake at 350 degrees F (175 degrees C) for about 45 minutes.

Nutrition Facts Per Serving:

- 316 calories

- protein 2.4g

- carbohydrates 60.5g

- fat 8.4g

- cholesterol 20.3mg

- sodium 97.9mg

Sarah's Applesauce

Prep: 10 mins

Cook: 20 mins

Total: 30 mins

Servings: 4

Yield: 4 servings

Ingredients

- 4 apples - peeled, cored and chopped

- ¾ cup water

- ¼ cup white sugar

- ½ teaspoon ground cinnamon

Instructions

• In a saucepan, combine apples, water, sugar, and cinnamon. Cover, and cook over medium heat for 15 to 20 minutes, or until apples are soft.

• Allow to cool, then mash with a fork or potato masher.

Nutrition Facts Per Serving:

• 121 calories

• protein 0.4g

• carbohydrates 31.8g

• fat 0.2g

• sodium 2.7mg

Chicken Quesadillas

Prep: 30 mins

Cook: 25 mins

Total: 55 mins

Servings: 20

Yield: 20 servings

Ingredients

• 1 pound skinless, boneless chicken breast, diced

• 1 (1.27 ounce) packet fajita seasoning

• 1 tablespoon vegetable oil

• 2 green bell peppers, chopped

• 2 red bell peppers, chopped

• 1 onion, chopped

• 10 (10 inch) flour tortillas

• 1 (8 ounce) package shredded Cheddar cheese

• 1 tablespoon bacon bits

• 1 (8 ounce) package shredded Monterey Jack cheese

Instructions

• Preheat the broiler. Grease a baking sheet.

• Toss the chicken with the fajita seasoning, then spread onto the baking sheet. Place under the broiler and cook until the chicken pieces are no longer pink in the center, about 5 minutes.

• Preheat oven to 350 degrees F (175 degrees C).

• Heat the oil in a large saucepan over medium heat. Stir in the green bell peppers, red bell peppers, onion, and chicken. Cook and stir until the vegetables have softened, about 10 minutes.

• Layer half of each tortilla with the chicken and vegetable mixture, then sprinkle with the Cheddar cheese, bacon bits, and Monterey Jack. Fold the tortillas in half and Place onto a baking sheet.

• Bake quesadillas in the preheated oven until the cheeses have melted, about 10 minutes.

Nutrition Facts Per Serving:

• 244 calories

• protein 13.7g

• carbohydrates 21.8g

• fat 11.3g

- cholesterol 34.9mg

- sodium 504.3mg

Prep: 5 mins

Cook: 15 mins

Total: 20 mins

Servings: 8

Yield: 4 cups

Ingredients

- ¼ cup butter

- 4 large tart apples - peeled, cored and sliced 1/4 inch thick

- 2 teaspoons cornstarch

- ½ cup cold water

- ½ cup brown sugar

- ½ teaspoon ground cinnamon

Instructions

• In a large skillet or saucepan, melt butter over medium heat; add apples. Cook, stirring constantly, until apples are almost tender, about 6 to 7 minutes.

• Dissolve cornstarch in water; add to skillet. Stir in brown sugar and cinnamon. Boil for 2 minutes, stirring occasionally. Remove from heat and serve warm.

Nutrition Facts Per Serving:

• 143 calories

• protein 0.4g

• carbohydrates 24.3g

• fat 5.9g

• cholesterol 15.3mg

• sodium 45mg

Bread and Celery Stuffing

Prep: 20 mins

Cook: 40 mins

Additional: 1 hr

Total: 2 hrs

Servings: 10

Yield: 10 servings

Ingredients

• 1 (1 pound) loaf sliced white bread

• ¾ cup butter or margarine

• 1 onion, chopped

• 4 stalks celery, chopped

• 2 teaspoons poultry seasoning

• salt and pepper to taste

• 1 cup chicken broth

Instructions

• Let bread slices air dry for 1 to 2 hours, then cut into cubes.

• In a Dutch oven, melt butter or margarine over medium heat. Cook onion and celery until soft. Season with poultry seasoning, salt, and pepper. Stir in bread cubes until evenly coated. Moisten with chicken broth; mix well.

• Chill, and use as a stuffing for turkey, or bake in a buttered casserole dish at 350 degrees F (175 degrees C) for 30 to 40 minutes.

Nutrition Facts Per Serving:

• 254 calories

• protein 4.4g

• carbohydrates 24.7g

• fat 15.5g

• cholesterol 36.6mg

• sodium 613.1mg

Blueberry Pie

Prep: 15 mins

Cook: 50 mins

Total: 1 hr 5 mins

Servings: 8

Yield: 1 pie

Ingredients

• ¾ cup white sugar

• 3 tablespoons cornstarch

• ¼ teaspoon salt

• ½ teaspoon ground cinnamon

• 4 cups fresh blueberries

• 1 recipe pastry for a 9 inch double crust pie

• 1 tablespoon butter

Instructions

• Preheat oven to 375 degrees F (190 degrees C).

• Mix sugar, cornstarch, salt, and cinnamon, and sprinkle over blueberries.

• Line pie dish with one pie crust. Pour berry mixture into the crust, and dot with butter. Cut remaining pastry into 1/2 - 3/4 inch wide strips, and make lattice top. Crimp and flute edges.

• Bake pie on lower shelf of oven for about 50 minutes, or until crust is golden brown.

Note:

• This recipe originally indicated an oven temperature of 425 degrees F (220 degrees C). It was revised to 375 degrees F (190 degrees C) based on reviews.

Nutrition Facts Per Serving:

• 366 calories

• protein 3.3g

• carbohydrates 52.6g

• fat 16.6g

• cholesterol 3.8mg

• sodium 317.7mg

Baked Ham and Cheese Party Sandwiches

Prep: 15 mins

Cook: 20 mins

Total: 35 mins

Servings: 24

Yield: 24 servings

Ingredients

• ¾ cup melted butter

• 1 ½ tablespoons Dijon mustard

• 1 ½ teaspoons Worcestershire sauce

• 1 ½ tablespoons poppy seeds

• 1 tablespoon dried minced onion

• 24 mini sandwich rolls

• 1 pound thinly sliced cooked deli ham

• 1 pound thinly sliced Swiss cheese

Instructions

• Preheat oven to 350 degrees F (175 degrees C). Grease a 9x13-inch baking dish.

• In a bowl, mix together butter, Dijon mustard, Worcestershire sauce, poppy seeds, and dried onion.

Separate the tops from bottoms of the rolls, and place the bottom pieces into the prepared baking dish. Layer about half the ham onto the rolls. Arrange the Swiss cheese over the ham, and top with remaining ham slices in a layer.

• Place the tops of the rolls onto the sandwiches. Pour the mustard mixture evenly over the rolls.

• Bake in the preheated oven until the rolls are lightly browned and the cheese has melted, about 20 minutes. Slice into individual rolls through the ham and cheese layers to serve.

Nutrition Facts Per Serving:

• 208 calories

• protein 9.8g

• carbohydrates 10.8g

• fat 14g

• cholesterol 43.4mg

• sodium 439.2mg

Apple Crisp

Prep: 10 mins

Cook: 40 mins

Additional: 10 mins

Total: 1 hr

Servings: 6

Yield: 1 8-inch square dish

Ingredients

• 2 ½ cups apples - peeled, cored, and sliced

• 1 cup sifted all-purpose flour

• 1 cup white sugar

• ½ teaspoon ground cinnamon

• ¼ teaspoon salt

• ½ cup butter, softened

Instructions

• Preheat oven to 375 degrees F (190 degrees C). Lightly grease an 8-inch square baking dish.

• Arrange apple slices evenly in prepared baking dish. Sift flour, sugar, cinnamon, and salt in a bowl. Cut in butter using a pastry blender or 2 knives until mixture resembles coarse cornmeal; sprinkle over apples.

• Bake in preheated oven until topping is golden, 40 to 45 minutes. Cool slightly before serving.

Note:

• Do not overmix the topping, and Never cream it. The topping should be gently cut into the butter so that the butter remains in small lumps. This will result in a light, crunchy topping for the apples. Also, in a pinch, you don't need to sift the dry ingredients. Just carefully stir them together until mixed (prior to adding the butter).

Nutrition Facts Per Serving:

• 365 calories

• protein 2.4g

• carbohydrates 55.7g

• fat 15.6g

• cholesterol 40.7mg

• sodium 206.7mg

Buffalo Chicken Dip

Prep: 5 mins

Cook: 40 mins

Total: 45 mins

Servings: 20

Yield: 5 cups

Ingredients

• 2 (10 ounce) cans chunk chicken, drained

• 2 (8 ounce) packages cream cheese, softened

• 1 cup Ranch dressing

• ¾ cup pepper sauce (such as Frank's Red Hot®)

• 1 ½ cups shredded Cheddar cheese

• 1 bunch celery, cleaned and cut into 4 inch pieces

• 1 (8 ounce) box chicken-flavored crackers

Instructions

• Heat chicken and hot sauce in a skillet over medium heat, until heated through. Stir in cream cheese and ranch dressing. Cook, stirring until well blended and warm.

• Mix in half of the shredded cheese, and transfer the mixture to a slow cooker. Sprinkle the remaining cheese over the top, cover, and cook on Low setting until hot and bubbly. Serve with celery sticks and crackers.

Nutrition Facts Per Serving:

• 284 calories

• protein 11.1g

• carbohydrates 8.6g

• fat 22.6g

• cholesterol 54.1mg

• sodium 551.8mg

Mom's Zucchini Bread

Prep: 20 mins

Cook: 1 hr

Additional: 20 mins

Total: 1 hr 40 mins

Servings: 24

Yield: 2 loaves

Ingredients

• 3 cups all-purpose flour

• 1 teaspoon salt

• 1 teaspoon baking soda

• 1 teaspoon baking powder

• 1 tablespoon ground cinnamon

• 3 eggs

• 1 cup vegetable oil

• 2 ¼ cups white sugar

• 3 teaspoons vanilla extract

• 2 cups grated zucchini

• 1 cup chopped walnuts

Instructions

• Grease and flour two 8 x 4 inch pans. Preheat oven to 325 degrees F (165 degrees C).

• Sift flour, salt, baking powder, soda, and cinnamon together in a bowl.

• Beat eggs, oil, vanilla, and sugar together in a large bowl. Add sifted ingredients to the creamed mixture, and beat well. Stir in zucchini and nuts until well combined. Pour batter into prepared pans.

• Bake for 40 to 60 minutes, or until tester inserted in the center comes out clean. Cool in pan on rack for 20 minutes. Remove bread from pan, and completely cool.

Nutrition Facts Per Serving:

• 255 calories

• protein 3.3g

- carbohydrates 32.1g

- fat 13.1g

- cholesterol 23.3mg

- sodium 179.8mg

Apple Strudel Muffins

Prep: 20 mins

Cook: 20 mins

Additional: 20 mins

Total: 1 hr

Servings: 12

Yield: 12 muffins

Ingredients

- 2 cups all-purpose flour

- 1 teaspoon baking powder

- ½ teaspoon baking soda

- ½ teaspoon salt

- ½ cup butter

- 1 cup white sugar

- 2 eggs

- 1 ¼ teaspoons vanilla

- 1 ½ cups chopped apples

- ⅓ cup packed brown sugar

- 1 tablespoon all-purpose flour

- ⅛ teaspoon ground cinnamon

- 1 tablespoon butter

Instructions

- Preheat oven to 375 degrees F (190 degrees C). Grease a 12 cup muffin pan.

- In a medium bowl, mix flour, baking powder, baking soda and salt.

- In a large bowl, beat together butter, sugar and eggs until smooth. Mix in vanilla. Stir in apples, and gradually blend in the flour mixture. Spoon the mixture into the prepared muffin pan.

• In a small bowl, mix brown sugar, flour and cinnamon. Cut in butter until mixture is like coarse crumbs. Sprinkle over tops of mixture in muffin pan.

• Bake 20 minutes in the preheated oven, or until a toothpick inserted in the center of a muffin comes out clean. Allow to sit 5 minutes before removing muffins from pan. Cool on a wire rack.

Nutrition Facts Per Serving:

• 264 calories

• protein 3.4g

• carbohydrates 41.4g

• fat 9.7g

• cholesterol 53.9mg

• sodium 254.6mg

Pesto Pasta

Prep: 5 mins

Additional: 10 mins

Total: 15 mins

Servings: 8

Yield: 8 servings

Ingredients

- ½ cup chopped onion

- 2 ½ tablespoons pesto

- 2 tablespoons olive oil

- 2 tablespoons grated Parmesan cheese

- 1 (16 ounce) package pasta

- salt to taste

- ground black pepper to taste

Instructions

- Cook pasta in a large pot of boiling water until done. Drain.

• Meanwhile, heat the oil in a frying pan over medium low heat. Add pesto, onion, and salt and pepper. Cook about five minutes, or until onions are soft.

• In a large bowl, mix pesto mixture into pasta. Stir in grated cheese. Serve.

Nutrition Facts Per Serving:

• 225 calories

• protein 7.8g

• carbohydrates 32g

• fat 7.2g

• cholesterol 43.5mg

• sodium 71.3mg

Homemade Apple Cider

Prep: 15 mins

Cook: 3 hrs 20 mins

Additional: 4 hrs

Total: 7 hrs 35 mins

Servings: 16

Yield: 1 gallon cider

Ingredients

• 10 apples, quartered

• ¾ cup white sugar

• 1 tablespoon ground cinnamon

• 1 tablespoon ground allspice

Instructions

• Place apples in a large stockpot and add enough water cover by at least 2 inches. Stir in sugar, cinnamon, and allspice. Bring to a boil. Boil, uncovered, for 1 hour. Cover pot, reduce heat, and simmer for 2 hours.

• Strain apple mixture though a fine mesh sieve. Discard solids. Drain cider again though a cheesecloth lined sieve. Refrigerate until cold.

Note

• Cider may be frozen for longer storage.

Nutrition Facts Per Serving:

• 83 calories

• protein 0.3g

• carbohydrates 21.9g

• fat 0.2g

• sodium 1.2mg

Chicken and Noodles

Prep: 10 mins

Cook: 30 mins

Total: 40 mins

Servings: 6

Yield: 6 servings

Ingredients

• 1 (26 ounce) can condensed cream of chicken soup

• 1 (10.75 ounce) can condensed cream of mushroom soup

• 3 (14.5 ounce) cans chicken broth

• 2 cups diced, cooked chicken breast meat

• 2 teaspoons onion powder

• 1 teaspoon seasoning salt

• ½ teaspoon garlic powder

• 2 (9 ounce) packages frozen egg noodles

Instructions

• In a large pot, mix the cream of chicken soup, cream of mushroom soup, chicken broth, and chicken meat.

• Season with onion powder, seasoning salt, and garlic powder. Bring to a boil, and stir in the noodles. Reduce heat to low, and simmer for 20 to 30 minutes.

Nutrition Facts Per Serving:

• 504 calories

• protein 27.4g

• carbohydrates 54.8g

• fat 19.6g

- cholesterol 98.7mg

- sodium 2355.6mg

Southern Pimento Cheese

Prep: 10 mins

Total: 10 mins

Servings: 12

Yield: 3 cups

Ingredients

- 2 cups shredded extra-sharp Cheddar cheese

- 8 ounces cream cheese, softened

- ½ cup mayonnaise

- ¼ teaspoon garlic powder

- ¼ teaspoon ground cayenne pepper (Optional)

- ¼ teaspoon onion powder

- 1 jalapeno pepper, seeded and minced (Optional)

- 1 (4 ounce) jar diced pimento, drained

• salt and black pepper to taste

Instructions

• Place the Cheddar cheese, cream cheese, mayonnaise, garlic powder, cayenne pepper, onion powder, minced jalapeno, and pimento into the large bowl of a mixer. Beat at medium speed, with paddle if possible, until thoroughly combined. Season to taste with salt and black pepper.

Nutrition Facts Per Serving:

• 208 calories

• protein 6.3g

• carbohydrates 2.1g

• fat 19.9g

• cholesterol 44.2mg

• sodium 229mg

Southern Pimento Cheese

Prep: 10 mins

Total: 10 mins

Servings: 12

Yield: 3 cups

Ingredients

• 2 cups shredded extra-sharp Cheddar cheese

• 8 ounces cream cheese, softened

• ½ cup mayonnaise

• ¼ teaspoon garlic powder

• ¼ teaspoon ground cayenne pepper (Optional)

• ¼ teaspoon onion powder

• 1 jalapeno pepper, seeded and minced (Optional)

• 1 (4 ounce) jar diced pimento, drained

• salt and black pepper to taste

Instructions

• Place the Cheddar cheese, cream cheese, mayonnaise, garlic powder, cayenne pepper, onion powder, minced jalapeno, and pimento into the large bowl of a mixer. Beat at medium speed, with paddle if possible, until thoroughly combined.

• Season to taste with salt and black pepper.

Nutrition Facts Per Serving:

• 208 calories

• protein 6.3g

• carbohydrates 2.1g

• fat 19.9g

• cholesterol 44.2mg

• sodium 229mg

Slow Cooker Stuffing

Prep: 25 mins

Cook: 8 hrs 55 mins

Total: 9 hrs 20 mins

Servings: 16

Yield: 16 servings

Ingredients

• 1 cup butter or margarine

• 2 cups chopped onion

• 2 cups chopped celery

• ¼ cup chopped fresh parsley

• 12 ounces sliced mushrooms

• 12 cups dry bread cubes

• 1 teaspoon poultry seasoning

• 1 ½ teaspoons dried sage

• 1 teaspoon dried thyme

• ½ teaspoon dried marjoram

• 1 ½ teaspoons salt

• ½ teaspoon ground black pepper

• 4 ½ cups chicken broth, or as needed

• 2 eggs, beaten

Instructions

• Melt butter or margarine in a skillet over medium heat. Cook onion, celery, mushroom, and parsley in butter, stirring frequently.

• Spoon cooked vegetables over bread cubes in a very large mixing bowl. Season with poultry seasoning, sage, thyme, marjoram, and salt and pepper. Pour in enough broth to moisten, and mix in eggs. Transfer mixture to slow cooker, and cover.

• Cook on High for 45 minutes, then reduce heat to Low, and cook for 4 to 8 hours.

Note

• To make the slow cooker stuffing in the oven, prepare as directed using the full amount of broth. Transfer to a 9x13 inch baking dish or other large casserole dish. Bake uncovered for 45 minutes to 1 hour at 350 degrees F (175 degrees C).

Nutrition Facts Per Serving:

• 197 calories

- protein 3.9g

- carbohydrates 16.6g

- fat 13.1g

- cholesterol 53.8mg

- sodium 501.7mg

Sarah's Rice Pilaf

Prep: 10 mins

Cook: 35 mins

Additional: 5 mins

Total: 50 mins

Servings: 4

Yield: 4 servings

Ingredients

- 2 tablespoons butter

- ½ cup orzo pasta

- ½ cup diced onion

• 2 cloves garlic, minced

• ½ cup uncooked white rice

• 2 cups chicken broth

Instructions

• Melt the butter in a lidded skillet over medium-low heat. Cook and stir orzo pasta until golden brown. Stir in onion and cook until onion becomes translucent, then add garlic and cook for 1 minute. Mix in the rice and chicken broth. Increase heat to high and bring to a boil.

• Reduce heat to medium-low, cover, and simmer until the rice is tender, and the liquid has been absorbed, 20 to 25 minutes. Remove from heat and let stand for 5 minutes, then fluff with a fork.

Nutrition Facts Per Serving:

• 244 calories

• protein 5.9g

• carbohydrates 40g

• fat 6.5g

• cholesterol 17.8mg

• sodium 524.3mg

Spiced Slow Cooker Applesauce

Prep: 10 mins

Cook: 6 hrs 30 mins

Total: 6 hrs 40 mins

Servings: 8

Yield: 8 servings

Ingredients

• 8 apples - peeled, cored, and thinly sliced

• ½ cup water

• ¾ cup packed brown sugar

• ½ teaspoon pumpkin pie spice

Instructions

• Combine the apples and water in a slow cooker; cook on Low for 6 to 8 hours. Stir in the brown sugar and pumpkin pie spice; continue cooking another 30 minutes.

Nutrition Facts Per Serving:

• 151 calories

• protein 0.4g

• carbohydrates 39.4g

• fat 0.2g

• sodium 7.7mg

Apple Bread

Prep: 20 mins

Cook: 1 hr 30 mins

Additional: 10 mins

Total: 2 hrs

Servings: 16

Yield: 2 loaves

Ingredients

- cooking spray

- 3 cups all-purpose flour

- 1 teaspoon baking soda

- 1 teaspoon salt

- 1 cup chopped walnuts (Optional)

- 3 cups apples - peeled, cored, and chopped

- 1 cup vegetable oil

- 2 cups white sugar

- 3 eggs, beaten

- 2 teaspoons ground cinnamon

Instructions

- Preheat oven to 300 degrees F (150 degrees C). Prepare 2 loaf pans (8 1/2x4 1/2-inch loaf pans) with cooking spray.

- Mix flour, baking soda, salt, walnuts, and apples in a large bowl. Whisk oil, sugar, eggs, and cinnamon together in a small bowl; add to flour mixture and mix until just moistened. Evenly divide mixture between prepared loaf pans.

• Bake in preheated oven until a toothpick inserted into the center comes out clean, about 90 minutes. Cool in the pans for 10 minutes before removing to cool completely on a wire rack.

Nutrition Facts Per Serving:

• 377 calories

• protein 4.8g

• carbohydrates 47.4g

• fat 19.6g

• cholesterol 34.9mg

• sodium 238mg

Apple Oatmeal Crisp

Prep: 20 mins

Cook: 40 mins

Total: 1 hr

Servings: 8

Yield: 1 - 8 inch square pan

Ingredients

• 1 cup brown sugar

• 1 cup rolled oats

• 1 cup all-purpose flour

• ½ cup butter, melted

• 3 cups apples - peeled, cored and chopped

• ½ cup white sugar

• 2 teaspoons ground cinnamon

Instructions

• Preheat oven to 350 degrees F (175 degrees C). Lightly grease an 8-inch square pan.

• In a large bowl, combine brown sugar, oats, flour and butter. Mix until crumbly. Place half of crumb mixture in pan. Spread the apples evenly over crumb mixture. Sprinkle with sugar and cinnamon and top with remaining crumb mixture.

• Bake in the preheated oven for 40 to 45 minutes, or until golden brown.

Nutrition Facts Per Serving:

• 376 calories

• protein 3.2g

• carbohydrates 65.2g

• fat 12.4g

• cholesterol 30.5mg

• sodium 90.9mg

Indian Style Basmati Rice

Prep: 10 mins

Cook: 25 mins

Additional: 10 mins

Total: 45 mins

Servings: 6

Yield: 6 servings

Ingredients

• 1 ½ cups basmati rice

• 2 tablespoons vegetable oil

• 1 (2 inch) piece cinnamon stick

• 2 pods green cardamom

• 2 whole cloves

• 1 tablespoon cumin seed

• 1 teaspoon salt, or to taste

• 2 ½ cups water

• 1 small onion, thinly sliced

Instructions

• Place rice into a bowl with enough water to cover. Set aside to soak for 20 minutes.

• Heat the oil in a large pot or saucepan over medium heat. Add the cinnamon stick, cardamom pods, cloves, and cumin seed. Cook and stir for about a minute, then add the onion to the pot.

• Saute the onion until a rich golden brown, about 10 minutes. Drain the water from the rice, and stir into the pot. Cook and stir the rice for a few minutes, until lightly toasted.

• Add salt and water to the pot, and bring to a boil. Cover, and reduce heat to low. Simmer for about 15 minutes, or until all of the water has been absorbed. Let stand for 5 minutes, then fluff with a fork before serving.

Nutrition Facts Per Serving:

• 216 calories

• protein 3.9g

• carbohydrates 38.9g

• fat 5.4g

• sodium 393.7mg

Crustless Cranberry Pie

Prep: 15 mins

Cook: 40 mins

Total: 55 mins

Servings: 8

Yield: 1 (9-inch) pie

Ingredients

• 1 cup all-purpose flour

• 1 cup white sugar

• ¼ teaspoon salt

• 2 cups cranberries

• ½ cup chopped walnuts

• ½ cup butter, melted

• 2 eggs

• 1 teaspoon almond extract

Instructions

• Preheat oven to 350 degrees F (175 degrees C). Grease one 9 inch pie pan.

• Combine the flour, sugar, and salt. Stir in the cranberries and the walnuts, and toss to coat. Stir in the butter, beaten eggs, and almond extract. If you are using frozen cranberries, the mixture will be very thick. Spread the batter into the prepared pan.

• Bake at 350 degrees F (175 degrees C) for 40 minutes, or until a wooden pick inserted near the center comes out clean. Serve warm with whipped cream or ice cream.

Nutrition Facts Per Serving:

• 335 calories

• protein 4.5g

• carbohydrates 41.4g

• fat 17.7g

• cholesterol 77mg

• sodium 172.9mg

Prep: 15 mins

Cook: 45 mins

Total: 1 hr

Servings: 6

Yield: 6 servings

Ingredients

• 5 cups peeled, cored, and sliced tart apples

• 2 teaspoons white sugar

• ½ teaspoon ground cinnamon

• 1 ½ cups brown sugar

• ¾ cup all-purpose flour

• ½ cup butter, softened

Instructions

• Preheat oven to 350 degrees F (175 degrees C).

• Place the apples into an ungreased 7x11-inch baking dish and sprinkle them with the sugar and cinnamon. Stir to combine thoroughly.

• In a bowl, mix together the brown sugar, flour, and softened butter until well combined; sprinkle over the apples.

• Bake in the preheated oven for until the apples are bubbling and the topping is lightly browned, 45 to 60 minutes. Serve hot.

Nutrition Facts Per Serving:

• 384 calories

• protein 2.1g

• carbohydrates 61.7g

• fat 15.7g

• cholesterol 40.7mg

• sodium 120.4mg

Tuna Fish Salad

Prep: 15 mins

Total: 15 mins

Servings: 4

Yield: 4 servings

Ingredients

- 1 (5 ounce) can tuna, drained

- 1 tablespoon chopped fresh parsley

- ¼ cup chopped celery

- ½ cup mayonnaise

- ½ teaspoon lemon juice

- ¼ cup chopped onion

- ¼ teaspoon garlic powder

- ⅛ teaspoon salt

- ⅛ teaspoon ground black pepper

- paprika to taste

Instructions

• In a large bowl, combine the tuna, celery, onion, mayonnaise, lemon juice, parsley, garlic powder, salt and pepper. Mix well and refrigerate until chilled. Sprinkle with paprika if desired.

Nutrition Facts Per Serving:

• 240 calories

• protein 8.5g

• carbohydrates 2.3g

• fat 22.1g

• cholesterol 19.9mg

• sodium 251.6mg

Blueberry Sour Cream Coffee Cake

Prep: 20 mins

Cook: 1 hr

Total: 1 hr 20 mins

Servings: 12

Yield: 1 - 9 inch Bundt cake

Ingredients

- 1 cup butter, softened

- 2 cups white sugar

- 2 eggs

- 1 cup sour cream

- 1 teaspoon vanilla extract

- 1 ⅝ cups all-purpose flour

- 1 teaspoon baking powder

- ¼ teaspoon salt

- 1 cup fresh or frozen blueberries

- ½ cup brown sugar

- 1 teaspoon ground cinnamon

- ½ cup chopped pecans

- 1 tablespoon confectioners' sugar for dusting

Instructions

• Preheat the oven to 350 degrees F (175 degrees C). Grease and flour a 9 inch Bundt pan.

• In a large bowl, cream together the butter and sugar until light and fluffy. Beat in the eggs one at a time, then stir in the sour cream and vanilla. Combine the flour, baking powder, and salt; stir into the batter just until blended. Fold in blueberries.

• Spoon half of the batter into the prepared pan. In a small bowl, stir together the brown sugar, cinnamon and pecans. Sprinkle half of this mixture over the batter in the pan. Spoon remaining batter over the top, and then sprinkle the remaining pecan mixture over. Use a knife or thin spatula to swirl the sugar layer into the cake.

• Bake for 55 to 60 minutes in the preheated oven, or until a knife inserted into the crown of the cake comes out clean. Cool in the pan over a wire rack. Invert onto a serving plate, and tap firmly to remove from the pan. Dust with confectioners' sugar just before serving.

Nutrition Facts Per Serving:

• 459 calories

- protein 4.1g

- carbohydrates 59.5g

- fat 24g

- cholesterol 80.1mg

- sodium 222.9mg

Turkey a la King

Prep: 10 mins

Cook: 15 mins

Total: 25 mins

Servings: 4

Yield: 4 servings

Ingredients

- 2 tablespoons butter

- 3 fresh mushrooms, sliced

- 1 tablespoon all-purpose flour

- 1 cup chicken broth

• ½ cup heavy cream

• 1 cup chopped cooked turkey

• ⅓ cup frozen peas, thawed

• salt and pepper to taste

Instructions

• In a large skillet over medium low heat, cook butter until golden brown. Saute mushrooms until tender.

• Stir in flour until smooth. Slowly whisk in chicken broth, and cook until slightly thickened. Stir in cream, turkey and peas. Reduce heat to low, and cook until thickened. Season with salt and pepper.

Nutrition Facts Per Serving:

• 233 calories

• protein 12.2g

• carbohydrates 4.5g

• fat 18.6g

• cholesterol 82.6mg

• sodium 91.5mg